Helping Hands
*Caregivers' Guide
for Drug-Exposed Infants*

Lisa M. Nelson
(425) 641-3347

Helping Hands
Caregivers' Guide for Drug-Exposed Infants

Barbara Drennen and Barbara Richards

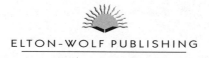

ELTON-WOLF PUBLISHING

Seattle • Los Angeles

Copyright © 2000 Barbara Drennen and Barbara Richards

All rights reserved.

Cover design, Sarah Watson
Text design, Paulette Eickman
Illustrator, Kathleen Dickson

No part of this book may be reproduced or utilized in any form or by any means, electronic or mechanical, including photocopying and recording, or by any information storage and retrieval system, without permission in writing from the author.

01 02 03 04 05   1 2 3 4 5

ISBN: 1-58783-005-1
Library of Congress Catalog Card Number: 00-108435

First Printing November 2000
Printed in Canada

Published by Elton-Wolf Publishing
Seattle, Washington

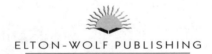

ELTON-WOLF PUBLISHING

2505 Second Avenue Suite 515   Seattle Washington 98121 (206) 748-0345
e-mail: info@elton-wolf.com   Internet: http://www.elton-wolf.com
Seattle • Los Angeles

About the Authors

Barbara Richards and Barbara Drennen are the cofounders and codirectors of the Pediatric Interim Care Center (PICC) located in Kent, Washington. The Center treats medically fragile newborns and infants who have been prenatally exposed to drugs. Both Barbara Richards and Barbara Drennen became foster mothers while in their twenties; they now have a combined fifty-six years of experience in infant care and have cared for over three hundred infants in their homes.

Barbara Richards previously served as the director of the Dun-Rovern Home for Exceptional Children in Nebraska from 1966–1984. She has been an advisory board member for the State Office of Mental Retardation in Nebraska, and has served on the Developmental Disabilities Task Force for the Medically Fragile and the Association for the Care of Children's Health. Presently, she serves on the Legislative Dependent Children's Study Group and is a member of the National Association for Female Executives, American Mothers, Inc., and the Washington State Governor's Task Force regarding infants born to drug-addicted mothers.

Barbara Drennen is a Washington State native who has managed the care of over a thousand newborns withdrawing from drugs. She has cared for more than 300 infants in her home as a foster parent and has adopted three children. She has been a member of the board of directors for her local school district, for the National Family Organization and for the Children's Therapy Center. She has also been a member of the Washington State Governor's Task Force for Medically Fragile Children and a juvenile court counselor. Drennen was named Washington State Mother of the Year in 1994, along with countless other local and national honors.

Both Richards and Drennen have been recipients of the prestigious Jefferson Award, and their work has been featured in *Family Circle* magazine, *British Nursing Magazine*, *Seattle Magazine*, and *American Mothers*. They have been featured on numerous national news programs, including "Dateline" on NBC, and "Eye on America" with CBS News anchorman Dan Rather.

Dedication

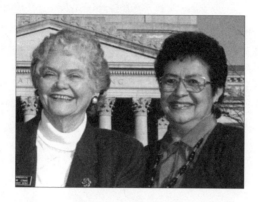

*Dedicated to
Washington State Representative, June Leonard and
Washington State Senator, Margarita Prentice*

*Our many thanks to two women
who cared enough to make a difference;*

*Women of great compassion who gave their time and commitment
to protect newborn infants prenatally exposed to
mothers' substance abuse and gave them a healthy start;*

*Women who fought to save the smallest victims who have been affected
by one of the country's greatest tragedies—drug addiction.*

We thank you and our babies thank you.

Acknowledgment

There is no way we can fully express the depths of our love, admiration and appreciation to our husbands Kenneth and Gary, and to our children for sharing their homes, their mothers, and their material blessings through the years. Without their continued support, it would have been impossible for us to establish and maintain a safe home for newborn infants in crisis.

Our heartfelt thanks to each and every one of you.

Preface

Together the Barbs watch over the safety of the babies

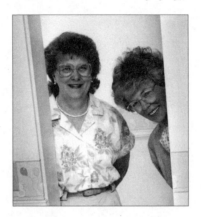

Without one another, Barb Drennen and Barb Richards couldn't have opened the Pediatric Interim Care Center (PICC) and maintained the operation that exists today. At times the challenges they faced seemed insurmountable. Had it not been for their undying love and need to protect the babies from society's ills, it is doubtful that they could have realized their dream.

TABLE OF CONTENTS

I: INTRODUCING THE PEDIATRIC INTERIM CARE CENTER ...... p. 5

II: GUIDE FOR INDIVIDUAL CAREGIVERS .... p. 15
   Common Threads .... p. 15
      Hypersensitivity to Stimuli .... p. 16
      Differences in Muscle Tone .... p. 17
      Sleeping Problems .... p. 17
      Feeding Problems .... p. 18
      Gastrointestinal Problems .... p. 18
   Therapeutic Handling .... p. 19
      Basic Principle 1: Swaddling .... p. 19
      Basic Principle 2: The C-Position .... p. 21
      Basic Principle 3: Head-to-Toe Movement .... p. 23
      Basic Principle 4: Vertical Rock .... p. 24
      Basic Principle 5: Clapping .... p. 25
      Basic Principle 6: Feeding .... p. 26
      Basic Principle 7: Controlling the Environment . p. 27
      Basic Principle 8: Introducing Stimuli .... p. 28

III: DRUG TYPES, SPECIFIC DRUGS, AND THEIR EFFECTS ..... p. 29
   The Effects on the Body of Each of these Drugs .... p. 30
      Stimulants .... p. 30
      Hallucinogens and Psychedelics .... p. 30
      Depressants .... p. 31
      Volatile Inhalants .... p. 31
      Opiates .... p. 32
      Psychotropics .... p. 32

Caregiving Techniques for Specific Drug Exposures ..... p. 33
    Cocaine or Crack ..... p. 33
    Amphetamines and Methamphetamines ..... p. 40
    Heroin and Methadone ..... p. 44
    Psychotropics ..... p. 50
    Alcohol Exposure ..... p. 52
A Caregiver's Continuing Responsibilities ..... p. 52

IV: RECORD KEEPING ..... p. 57
  Central Nervous System Disturbances ..... p. 59
    Crying ..... p. 59
    Sleep ..... p. 60
    Moro Reflex ..... p. 60
    Tremors ..... p. 61
    Increased Muscle Tone ..... p. 61
    Excoriation ..... p. 62
    Myoclonic Jerks ..... p. 62
    Convulsions/Seizures ..... p. 62
  Metabolic, Vasomotor, and Respiratory Disturbances .. p. 63
    Sweating ..... p. 63
    Fever ..... p. 63
    Frequent Yawning ..... p. 63
    Mottling ..... p. 63
    Nasal Stuffiness ..... p. 64
    Sneezing ..... p. 64
    Nasal Flaring ..... p. 64
    Respiratory Rate ..... p. 64

Gastrointestinal Disturbances .... p. 64
    Frantic or Disorganized Suck .... p. 64
    Excessive Sucking .... p. 65
    Flatus (Gas) .... p. 65
    Poor Feeding .... p. 65
    Regurgitation .... p. 65
    Projectile Vomiting .... p. 65
    Loose Stools .... p. 66
    Water-Ring Stools .... p. 66
    Watery Stools .... p. 66
    Neonatal Abstinence Scoring System .... p. 67

V: DEALING WITH DRUG-DEPENDENT MOTHERS .... p. 69
    Generalizations that may apply to
    Drug-Abusing Mothers .... p. 70
    Chances of Staying Drug-Free .... p. 71
    Feelings of Guilt and Embarrassment .... p. 71
    Lying about Behavior .... p. 72
    Dangerous Behavior .... p. 73
    Training in Maternal Skills .... p. 73
    Urging against Breast-feeding .... p. 74

VI: CONVERSATIONS WITH PEDIATRICIANS
AND CONCLUSION .... p. 77
    Dr. Peyton Gaunt .... p. 78
    Dr. David Woodrum .... p. 80
    Dr. Alvin Novack .... p. 85
    Conclusion .... p. 88

GLOSSARY .... p. 89

I

Introducing the Pediatric Interim Care Center

Over the past ten years, the Pediatric Interim Care Center (PICC) has been the step between hospital and home for more than 1,000 Washington State babies—babies who have been exposed to illegal or prescription drugs before birth and now must go through withdrawal. It's a very tough way for these beautiful babies to start their lives, so the care center is designed to meet their every need. The focus of the center is on getting the babies clean and giving them a chance to thrive.

The center has a homelike environment, is spotlessly clean, and is well adapted to taking care of newborns who don't need the intensive medical services of hospitals. What the babies do get is loving attention, close observation, and devoted people to help them through their withdrawal from drugs. The babies' rooms are quiet, subdued and decorated in soft colors, which are soothing to the infants. It's a matter of respect that the babies are clean at all times, that their rooms are immaculate and that they are handled in a caring, loving, and therapeutic way. There is a "dark room," a place with almost no sensory stimuli, for infants going through severe withdrawal. Other rooms are more brightly lit and have more decorations—these are for babies who are past the worst of their withdrawal symptoms and can tolerate more stimuli. There also are rooms for family members to stay near their infants.

You can't know any of this from outside the building. If you were to visit the center, located in the heart of Kent, Washington, you might think you had arrived at a suite of physicians' offices. The care center is a one-story, brick building that has the anonymous look of thousands of other respectable, quiet buildings in thousands of other towns and cities. Once inside, you see teddy bears and other stuffed animals, colorful toys, a few paintings, a few brochures, and chairs and sofas that make the room look more like a home than a front office. We're fortunate to have found this place because we can hardly imagine a better one to answer the needs of the babies we care for.

"We" are Barbara Drennen and Barbara Richards, the cofounders and codirectors of the Pediatric Interim Care Center. We oversee more than fifty staff members and more than 200 volunteers, and direct the babies' care in consultation with physicians and other medical professionals. Over the years, the center has received millions of dollars of donated goods and services, without which this work could not continue. The center runs partially on state funds, but primarily on the dedicated service of volunteers, board members, and staff. Whereas hospital care costs $2,500 per day, the costs of the Pediatric Interim Care Center remain at about $145 per day. We estimate that the care center has saved the state of Washington $18 million over the last ten years, dollars that would have been spent on unnecessary hospital care for these special babies.

We did not plan to become specialists in neonatal care for drug-exposed babies. We both became foster mothers in our early twenties, and with the support and partnership of our husbands, have nurtured foster children over a combined fifty-six years of care. We had handled many tough situations. But then something changed, and we both noticed it.

The year was 1985. Each of us was deeply involved in providing foster care in our homes. In addition to our own biological children, we had taken in hundreds of foster children and considered ourselves experts in the challenges that any foster parent faces. In fact, we both had specialized in caring for children with medical problems—hundreds of premature infants and medically fragile children. But we both became perplexed as more and more of the infants assigned to us showed the distressed (and distressing) symptoms of prenatal drug exposure.

These babies were more than fussy; they were inconsolable. If you opened their blankets to cool them on a hot summer's day, they screamed. If you turned on the fan, they screamed louder. They trembled, they cried, and they wouldn't be comforted. All the techniques that usually worked to quiet a fussy infant failed with these babies. If you bounced them to music, took them for a ride in the car, held them close, or spoke in a special voice, they only got worse. They were extremely difficult to feed. Their little bodies jerked as they slept. And nothing seemed to help.

About this time, we began putting our heads together as we handled one of the toughest assignments in all of foster care: twenty-four-hour home care for two children on respirators. It was more than a full-time job, requiring shifts of nurses coming in and out of our homes, maintaining intricate life-support equipment, and handling emergencies fairly regularly. We shared nurses, advice, information, and support with one another and became fast friends, as well as each other's consultant in working with drug-affected babies.

We shared a concern over the babies who were especially challenging due to their drug exposure—the ones who didn't respond to any of the normal calming techniques. We started trying techniques we had learned in caring for neurologically damaged infants—those who can't handle normal sensory input —and found that these techniques worked best with the challenging babies. We found other ways as well to get the babies to eat, to sleep, and to respond. Gradually, a regimen for care of drug-exposed babies came together in our minds and our practice.

We were also aware of increased numbers of premature (twenty-four weeks of gestation) infants—spontaneous deliveries from mothers addicted to cocaine. We saw hospital neonatal units overloaded with infants too fragile to go home. And we saw doctors working hard to help these little ones survive, only to have to send them into foster care before they were quite ready. The foster-care system at that time was in great need of homes for infants who clearly needed special care. It was a time of deep concern for the medical communities at large and especially the foster-care system.

We began to focus all of our energies on confronting the problem: What are the most effective forms of nurture for the drug-exposed infant? Focusing on the babies made us determined and we felt compelled to speak up to authority. We first approached the Washington State Department of Social and Health Services (DSHS) about this worsening problem. To our amazement, departmental staff asked us to do short-term medical-receiving care for drug-exposed infants in our homes. We would take the babies for about three months, bring them through the critical early withdrawal-and-adjustment phase, and get them healthy enough to be placed in regular homes. Clearly, we had established our credibility in this field of care, where there were few experts. But this small start at tackling the problem was far less than what everyone who knew about it agreed was needed. Several physicians asked us if we could provide services on a larger scale for these kinds of babies.

Despite our more than twenty years each of caring for medically fragile children and an abundance of hands-on medical knowledge, we had no formal medical training. If we were going to move to a larger scale of service, we both knew we needed to know more. We looked for classes all over the country and researched how other states were dealing with the problem.

We went to New York City to visit Mother Hale's Center in Harlem, the only facility we could find specifically licensed to provide care for drug-exposed children. Impressed as we were with Mother Hale—an inexhaustible woman with amazing determination—we found her caregiving techniques to be very similar to those we were already using in our own homes. Furthermore, the children under her care were older than ours and stayed in care for three to four years. We thought the greatest emphasis should be on the newborn, and we were convinced that the newborns' stay in special care should be only long enough to complete the withdrawal process. When it was medically safe, they should return to their families or go into foster care or adoption. We thought longer-term specialized care could easily lead to institutionalization, and we deeply believed that this outcome did not serve the best interests of any child.

We went to seminars, gleaning information. The more we searched, the more it became clear to us that nobody really knew how to deal with the problems drug-exposed infants presented. Even an expert pediatrician at Children's Hospital in Seattle told us, "You know as much as we do, and we must continue to learn together."

The care of drug-exposed infants became our mission. We designed an interim care center, where babies could be safely nurtured during the critical early weeks of life. Only in such a place, it seemed, could the babies be medically supervised and properly handled. And caregivers could learn how to handle these babies once they went home.

As needed as it was, the center we envisioned proved to be a hard political sell. It meant getting funding and support for something new, something untried. We made trip after trip to Olympia, the state capital to meet with the staff at DSHS, and often returned home frustrated.

Eventually, legislators—the real makers of policy and providers of funding—became involved. They were hearing from their constituents about the tremendous need to protect drug-exposed babies, and they came to our aid in making a case for an interim care center. The need became so obvious our proposal finally prevailed. With funding authorized directly from the legislature, and after two years of preparation, in 1990 we opened the door of the Pediatric Interim Care Center. We decided to divide the main duties of the center: Richards handling the business along with the volunteer program, Drennen managing all infant care and supervising nursing and social work. Drennen worked closely with the medical directors, Dr. Peyton Gaunt and Dr. Melvin Morse. We insisted on the word *interim* in the name so that everyone would know that this was a short-stay facility. It was not a hospital nor was it like any foster-care home, though it resembled both. It was the first center of its kind in the United States and remains through 2000 the only such center nationally.

In the ten plus years that we have operated the center, more than 1,000 babies have been lovingly and safely shepherded through the crisis of drug withdrawal. On any day, you can walk into the quiet, pastel rooms and see the babies in their cribs. They are not frantic. They are not screaming and jerking. In fact, there isn't much crying in the rooms. Many hands hold and feed the babies—a multitude of trained hands that know the techniques which make an amazing difference.

The drugs have changed. The crack and cocaine epidemic that spurred the creation of the center peaked in the 1980s, but the problem didn't go away. The 1990s brought more babies withdrawing from heroin and methadone. And now, early in a new century, we've seen a wave of infants exposed to methamphetamines and even more poly-substance abuse.

The babies who came in the center's early days are preteens now, and we are seeing some mothers return multiple times. We have kept track of many of the infants and their mothers, which leads us to say the one thing we know for sure: Drug-exposed infants can overcome their early problems and do well. The key to that success is the caregiver—a caregiver who is informed and prepared to provide the special techniques that we know will work.

The care starts the moment the baby arrives at the care center from the hospital. As you pass through an always-locked door into the hallway, you will probably hear a bit of crying from one or more of the fifteen babies, whose ages range from two hours to about thirty days. But it will be more like the crying sounds you expect to hear from an infant than the desperate crying or the "cat cry" you hear from an infant in withdrawal from drugs. That's because, as soon as we receive a drug-exposed infant from the birthing hospital, we begin the special care techniques described in this book.

We place three babies in each room, and we keep the lights low. You'll see a rocking chair, in addition to cribs, and in several rooms you'll see an adult—either a staff member or a volunteer. That person will be holding a swaddled baby. In other rooms you'll see peacefully sleeping babies and, on the doors of some rooms, a sign that says this baby needs complete isolation—NO VISITORS. These babies, though damaged by in utero drug exposure, are not doomed to living as severely handicapped adults. They are usually at least as intelligent as other newborns, and they can be productive citizens if they receive the kind of nurture they are entitled to.

When babies arrive at the center, they can look like little old people because of the difficulties they've experienced before birth. They may be wrinkled, with a sad look, or a severe frown between their eyes. Then, with loving handling, they begin to soften and look like an infant should. They begin to put on weight and begin to tolerate being cuddled. After about a month, the babies go home. High stress will be their lifelong enemy, but these babies are intelligent and can learn how to manage themselves in their environments. They can have healthy, normal lives once the drugs are out of their systems. That's why the care center exists—to provide a medically safe place for drug-affected infants, an interim step between hospital and home. It's a place where families can learn how to handle and care for their children.

Over the years, we have worked with wonderful, dedicated caregivers. When the babies leave the care center, twenty percent go home with parents, fifty-five percent go home with other relatives, and another twenty-five percent go into foster care. We have the babies for about thirty days; caregivers have them for many years and do the important job of helping the children thrive and develop into productive, successful citizens.

II

Guide for Individual Caregivers

COMMON THREADS

Over the last decade, the number of drug-affected infants has been growing. Studies at the University of Washington and the National Association for Perinatal Addiction Research (Chicago) conclude that as many as one-in-ten babies born in this country's urban centers suffers some degree of drug exposure. Few of those babies are ever diagnosed or referred for special care. Because the amount of time that mothers and babies spend in the hospital has shortened, the infants' symptoms are less likely to be recognized. It may be days, or even weeks, before an infant begins to go through withdrawal and starts to show the tremors, jerks, irritability, and other signs of drug exposure. By that time, the baby has left the hospital.

When the symptoms do hit, the situation can spiral out of control. Often, the baby is in the care of a parent who is undergoing the stress of his or her own drug addiction. If the baby is in an out-of-home placement, the relative, foster parent, or adoptive parent may not know or even suspect that drug exposure is the cause of the problems. The baby becomes extremely fussy and difficult to calm. He or she seems to reject the caregiver, arching away or screaming when the caregiver tries to hold the baby and give comfort. The infant rejects the bottle and it is almost impossible to feed more than a tiny amount. Sleep is occasional and brief. There may be constant diarrhea or constipation and gassiness. And the more the caregiver tries to help, the worse it seems to get. It's a scenario that can easily lead to frustration for the caregiver or failure to thrive for the baby.

The nature and timing of symptoms depend on a number of factors: (1) the drug to which the baby was exposed; (2) how the baby metabolizes the drug; and (3) the baby's own temperament and tolerance. We will deal with each of these factors at some length later, but first, here are the characteristics that drug-exposed babies have in common, though certainly no two are exactly alike.

Hypersensitivity to Stimuli

This trait is common to all drug-exposed infants. Almost everything is uncomfortable for them. They have little tolerance for light, bright colors, the touch of hands, loud music or voices. Even the act of swallowing formula can be overstimulating and make the baby frantic. It helps to know that the babies are not rejecting you when they recoil from touch. It's just that human closeness can be too stimulating, too distressing and uncomfortable. So are bright lights (particularly overhead light), music, talking, and cooing, bouncing and erratic movement. Even the sight of a face may be so intense that the baby involuntarily avoids eye contact.

However, this hypersensitivity to stimuli does not mean that drug-exposed babies should be left untouched in a dark room. What these babies need is protection from the overstimulation that can increase their distress. They need to have stimulation introduced more slowly and carefully than we normally do with a baby who has greater natural tolerance.

Differences in Muscle Tone

Tone is most easily understood as the degree of stiffness in the baby's muscles. Depending on the specific drug or drugs affecting them, the babies may be unusually limp or they may have a high degree of stiffness, particularly in the neck and limbs, or they may have a mixed tone—stiffness that comes and goes.

Underlying the stiffness of a baby in withdrawal from drugs is the baby's desperate attempt to control its body. The baby is feeling out of control because he or she may be experiencing tremors, jerking, and other feelings of distress. The tensing of muscles is a sign of trying to control those uncomfortable sensations.

It's easy to misread the real message of a baby with stiff muscle tone. The tense neck muscles seem like the baby is trying to lift its head. We've seen newborns with such high tone that they can lift their heads right off the mattress. It can seem that the baby is unusually strong rather than drug-affected. Their legs may be so tense that they seem to be trying to stand. In reality, the baby is fighting—and fighting hard—to control tremors and other internal discomforts.

Sleeping Problems

Again, the exact nature of the problems you see will depend on the drug and the degree of exposure. But, generally speaking, in the early days of withdrawal, drug-exposed infants do not sleep well. At times, their sleep is fitful and disturbed. They may have a difficult time falling asleep, or they may be so lethargic they can barely rouse to feed.

Feeding Problems

The greatest immediate danger facing some drug-exposed infants is failure to thrive. They use a tremendous amount of energy reacting to the environment and trying to control their bodies. At the same time, they face great difficulties that keep them from getting enough to eat. You might see disorganized sucking, rejection of the bottle after a small amount of feeding, inability to close their mouths around the nipple, fussiness, stomach cramps, lethargy and drowsing during feeding.

Gastrointestinal Problems

Some of the irritability we see in drug-exposed infants may be tied to gastrointestinal distress. Depending on the drugs affecting them, the babies may have watery stools, explosive diarrhea, irritated or scratched buttocks, gas, or constipation.

Without proper handling, these problems can become extremely dangerous. The more distressed the baby becomes, the more the gastrointestinal problems increase. The more the problems increase, the more distressed the baby becomes. The cycle repeats. Especially in the case of those infants with explosive or extreme diarrhea, the problems can quickly threaten their health—and even their lives. Out-of-control diarrhea can rip the fragile lining of an infant's intestine, requiring surgery or potentially causing death.

Fortunately, gastrointestinal problems can be controlled if the cycle of stress is broken. That is the goal of therapeutic handling: to reduce stimuli and reduce stress.

THERAPEUTIC HANDLING

It's not necessary for drug-exposed infants to cry for hours on end. They need not be too frantic to suck or too lethargic to complete a feeding. They don't have to claw the air with frantic, out-of-control limbs. They don't have to suffer. The key is therapeutic handling. We know it works because we have seen it work hundreds of times with the most severely affected drug-exposed infants.

Each type of drug exposure—like alcohol, cocaine, or heroin—presents a somewhat different challenge for caregivers. We'll discuss them each in detail in the following sections. But the basic principles of therapeutic handling are the same for all these infants.

Basic Principle 1: Swaddling

Drug-exposed infants cannot do three things simultaneously. They cannot control their bodies, breathe, and suck at the same time. If they are constantly focused on trying to control the discomfort in their bodies, they cannot focus on feeding and sleeping. We cannot breathe, eat, or sleep for them, but we can control their bodies for them. We do that by swaddling—wrapping them snugly to control their movements and provide comfort.

It is amazing how quickly distressed babies will get calm when swaddled. We can only imagine what a relief it must be for them to let go of the constant stiffening of their muscles. By swaddling and curling such babies, you help them begin to relax, eat, sleep, and respond. Swaddling helps control the baby's jerks and tremors; the security of swaddling gives their muscles a much-needed rest.

The best blanket for swaddling is lightweight and somewhat stretchy. At our center, we use lightweight cotton-thermal receiving blankets, which have the advantage of holding the swaddle and reducing the infant's constant tremors.

Swaddling needs to be snug, as shown in the illustration below. Fold the blanket in an offset triangle pointing downward. Tightly wrap the left corner over the baby's arms. Bring the bottom corner of the blanket up over the baby's legs and torso. Complete the swaddle by wrapping the right corner tightly around the baby's body. (A tight wrap prevents the baby's hands from pulling loose and scratching the face.) A properly swaddled baby should feel like a snug, little package in your arms. During the first month of life, drug-exposed infants should be swaddled the majority of the time.

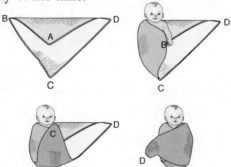

Basic Principle 2: The C-Position

To increase the swaddled infant's sense of control and relaxation, hold the body firmly and curl the head and legs around into a C, as shown here.

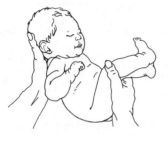

DO
A C-position is chin down resting near chest, arms forward, back is rounded slightly, legs are slightly bent in an upward position.

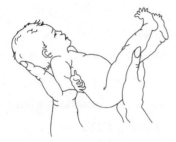

DON'T
Infant is working hard to control his own body by stiffening the back, arms, and legs. In doing this, he is increasing his body tone and burning precious calories he needs to grow.

If being held next to you is too stimulating and the baby's distress continues, you can turn the baby away from you and curl him or her into a C-position over your arm.

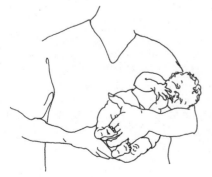

C-POSITION FACING OUT
Place your infant in C-hold with chin down, legs up, arms forward with back rounded forward. Face the baby away from your body. This hold is good for infants with increased tone using your body to break the baby's tendency to arch backward by molding his or her body forward.

When you lay the infant down, maintain the C-curl with the infant on his or her side. Do not lay the baby face down, and make sure there are no loose blankets, pillows, or toys in the crib that could obstruct breathing. Then wrap a blanket into a firm ring and encircle the baby's body to maintain the C-position. It is very important to have either a blanket roll surrounding the infant or a wedge up against the body so that the baby remains on his or her side at all times and does not roll onto the stomach.

At our care center, we use the side position because infants in the early days of withdrawal have such difficulty sleeping. The sideline C-position helps them feel more secure and relieves cramping and other gastrointestinal distress they may be feeling. As withdrawal symptoms diminish, you can introduce the back-sleeping position recommended by the Academy of Pediatrics to reduce the risk of sudden infant-death syndrome (SIDS).

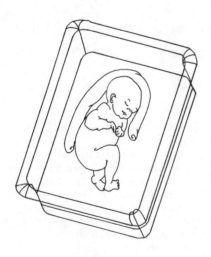

DO
Infant in sideline C-position in bed with rolled ring snugly around upper body and head.

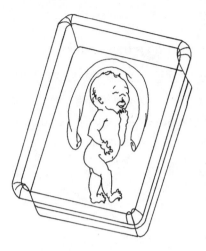

DON'T
Infant is stressed trying to control body and is burning calories. Notice the head is tilted back, the legs are extended at full length, and the back is vertically straight with a slight arch.

Basic Principle 3: Head-to-Toe Movement

For the drug-exposed infant, traditional techniques for quieting a fussy baby just don't work. Common techniques like back-and-forth rocking and bouncing your infant are not recommended. These motions are jarring to a drug-affected baby's nervous system.

Instead, sway slowly and rhythmically, with the baby swaddled and firmly held in a C-position. Calming movements should always follow a line from head to toe.

If the baby is still fussy when held against your body, you can turn him or her away from you, curled in a C-position over your arm. Then sway from side to side as the baby faces a blank floor or wall. Keep your movements slow and rhythmic. Notice again that the calming movement follows a line from head to toe.

Basic Principle 4: Vertical Rock

When you are holding a baby who is frantic and very hard to calm, you can maintain a C-hold directly in front of you, with the infant two inches away from your body and facing away from you. Then, slowly and rhythmically move the baby up and down. The head-to-toe movement is soothing to the baby's neurological system, as is keeping the baby away from your body.

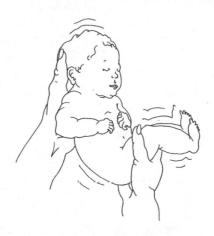

VERTICAL ROCK
When an infant is frantic and hard to calm, hold the baby as little as two inches from your body and rhythmically rock up and down slowly. When doing the vertical movements, make sure your baby is in a C-position and you have a tight grip on the baby. Three or four up-and-down movements generally will be enough, then pull the baby back into your body and hold snugly and sway from side to side rhythmically.

Basic Principle 5: Clapping

While you're swaying, another technique can help the baby relax: clapping. Cup your hand and clap slowly and rhythmically on the baby's diapered and blanketed bottom. Clap to the beat of your heart; you will feel the baby's muscles relax. The air pocket you clap with is very soothing and you can feel the baby soften and he may go into a deep sleep. Clapping can be very comforting for many babies, but, for some especially hypersensitive infants, this mode of calming is overstimulating.

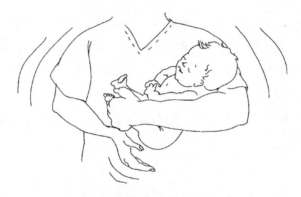

CLAP AND SWAY TO CALM INFANT
When trying to calm your infant, hold him or her in a tight C-position with chin down to chest, arms to the center of the body, legs bent slightly and pulled into the body. Cup hand and clap infants diapered bottom, clapping to the beat of the heart. While clapping the infant's bottom sway from side to side rhythmically, swaying from the knees rather than from the hips. This method will calm the baby, relaxing tight muscles, therefore allowing your baby to go into a deep sleep.

Basic Principle 6: Feeding

Babies withdrawing from opiates suck frantically, but it is hard for them to take in enough formula. Their stress levels are so high that they simply cannot organize an effective suck without help. The key to feeding is to get the baby to relax enough to suck. Always feed in a low-stimulus environment—no bright light, music, noise, fans, or other distractions. And make sure the baby is snugly swaddled and in the tight C-position.

Now the challenge is to get the baby to close his or her mouth around the nipple. With your hand holding the bottle, support the baby's chin with your index finger. With your arm holding the baby, increase the curl, wrapping the baby's body around into a tight C until you see the mouth close. By controlling the infant's body in this way, you allow him or her to relax and suck.

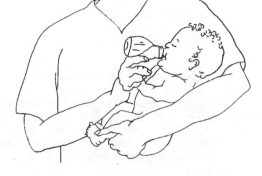

FEEDING POSITION
When feeding your baby, it will be necessary to control your baby's body so he or she can concentrate on nippling his or her formula. Your infant will not be able to close his or her mouth around the nipple without your support. The support will come in the C-position, hands forward to the chest, legs up and chin down and forward. The infant can do two things at once—breathe and suck or breathe and control his or her body, we cannot breathe or suck for the baby, but we can control his body so your baby can close his or her mouth around the nipple and suckle appropriately.

Basic Principle 7: Controlling the Environment

In order for therapeutic handling to be effective, babies need a calm, quiet environment. Loud or jarring noises increase their distress, so it's best to turn down the music and TV and discourage loud talking within the infant's earshot. Also, in the first weeks of withdrawal, overhead lights can be overstimulating. Light from a table lamp is more soothing.

Caregivers are the most important part of the baby's environment. Your calming presence and soothing ways are essential elements in the baby's recovery and health. The drug-exposed baby responds to the quiet voice; slow, smooth, deliberate movements; and calm handling. If you're feeling stressed or hurried, it's fine to stop for a few seconds, take a deep breath, slow down, and soften your voice before you approach the baby. If both you and the baby are stressed, it's also fine to let someone calmer take over the care for a while.

When babies show signs of overstimulation, it's best to minimize handling and protect them from situations where they are passed from lap to lap. Family and friends will understand that the infant has a hard time tolerating stimulation and needs some quiet time.

Basic Principle 8: Introducing Stimuli

All babies need stimulation for healthy development. With the drug-exposed infant, stimulation can be introduced in small doses as the baby's stress level allows. Since no two drug-exposed infants are exactly alike, neither are their tolerances or their timetables. Introducing stimuli is largely a matter of learning to "read" each baby and his or her responses.

It's best to go slowly and change the environment a little at a time. See first how the baby responds if the swaddling blanket is loosened. You can try gentle rocking and talking. If the baby begins showing signs of stress, like fussiness or stiffening of limbs, return to your therapeutic-handling techniques for a while longer. Early signs of overstimulation are yawning, sneezing, or hiccuping. They'll tell you that the baby needs some quiet time. This is an area where patience pays dividends. In time you'll find that the baby who once arched away will respond to you in a much more positive way.

III

Drug Types, Specific Drugs, and Their Effects

As we have said, the effects on infants of each type of drug are different. As you prepare for caring for drug-exposed babies, it will be helpful for you to know categories of drugs (like *stimulants*) and specific drug names (like *amphetamines*). We offer here a drug primer. Later, we'll explain how care procedures differ with different drugs. Unfortunately, however, the popularity of the drugs on the street change rapidly. So, some of what we tell you here will be changing over time.

This chart shows the category names and a few of the drugs that are classified within each:

CATEGORY NAME	SPECIFIC DRUGS
stimulants	amphetamines, cocaine, crack, tobacco
hallucinogens & psychedelics	marijuana, LSD, PCP, peyote/mescaline
depressants	alcohol, barbiturates, tranquilizers, quaaludes
volatile inhalants (or deliriants)	glue, nail polish remover, gasoline
opiates (or narcotic analgesics)	methadone, opium, heroin
psychotropics (or prescription drugs for psychiatric disorders)	haloperidol, chlorpromazine, thioridazine

THE EFFECTS ON THE BODY OF EACH OF THESE DRUGS

Stimulants

Stimulants increase activity of the heart and provide an overall sense of well-being, at least temporarily.

Amphetamines and Methamphetamines are manufactured chemicals that act similarly to adrenaline, the body's natural energy enhancer, speeding up several of the body's processes. Users take amphetamines orally; they smoke *methamphetamines*, which come in the form of crystals.

Cocaine and Crack are essentially the same—cocaine being a white powder and crack a solid substance that makes a cracking sound when smoked.

Tobacco is a plant in the nightshade family, which, when smoked, initially acts as a stimulant but, when taken in large doses, depresses body functions.

Hallucinogens and Psychedelics

Hallucinogens and psychedelics excite the brain, with the result that the user hallucinates, has mood changes, or even experiences short-term insanity.

Marijuana, made from the leaves of the cannabis plant, alters the mood of the user when he or she smokes, drinks (in a tea), or eats it. A stronger form of marijuana is hashish.

LSD is an acid (lysergic acid diethylamide) that is colorless, tasteless, and odorless but, when swallowed, acts on the brain to produce visions and other strange mental states.

PCP, another mind-altering substance, is one of the derivatives of phencyclidine, pharmacologically a very complex drug.

Peyote and Mescaline are similar in their ability to alter one's perception of things in the world. Peyote comes from a cactus; mescaline, when sold on the street, is a white crystal.

Note: All five of the drugs listed above have legitimate medical and/or religious uses.

Depressants

Depressants act on the central nervous system to produce both euphoria and drowsiness.

Alcohol increases the body's metabolic rate but also sedates and intoxicates, resulting in disorientation, mood swings, and slurred speech. Long-term effects include liver, brain, and heart damage.

Barbiturates, such as phenobarbital and nembutal, induce sleep by depressing the breathing rate, blood pressure, and temperature.

Tranquilizers, such as diazepam (Valium) and acetaminophen, slow down the central nervous system

Quaaludes are non-barbiturate sedatives, acting on a different part of the nervous system to induce relaxation and perhaps to lower sexual inhibition.

Note: Each of these drugs also has legal medical uses.

Volatile Inhalants (or Deliriants)

Volatile inhalants alter the mind.

Glue, nail polish remover, and gasoline are among solvent-based substances that give off fumes that can be in and produce a "high," a feeling of euphoria in the user.

Opiates (or Narcotic Analgesics)

Opiates reduce the sensation of pain and induce a feeling of well-being.

Methadone is a synthetic substance that produces a sense of well-being or euphoria, similar to heroin. It was developed as a substitute for heroin and morphine and is highly addictive.

Opium comes from a poppy. The smoke produced when it burns is inhaled to produce euphoria, though it can also be drunk.

Heroin was first produced by The Bayer Company (aspirin manufacturer) as a derivative of *morphine*, both powerful painkillers.

Psychotropics (or Prescription Drugs for Psychiatric Disorders)

Psychotropics (or prescription drugs for psychiatric disorders) are used to treat emotional, mental, and metabolic disorders.

Haloperidol is prescribed to control tics and symptoms of Tourette's syndrome and to treat severe behavior problems in children.

Chlorpromazine is used in treating migraine headaches and Huntington's disease.

Thioridazine (also known as Mellaril) is prescribed for depression, anxiety, sleep disturbances, and severe behavior problems in children.

CAREGIVING TECHNIQUES FOR SPECIFIC DRUG EXPOSURES
Cocaine or Crack (Stimulants)

The typical cocaine-exposed infant is prematurely born—under thirty-seven weeks gestation. The baby may be even smaller than a healthy infant of that gestation, but he or she will seem to be remarkably healthy: pink, soft, and cuddly. There will be no signs of tremor or any other withdrawal symptoms. In fact, the only way anyone can verify that the baby has been exposed in utero to cocaine is through what is called a tox screen—a urine test that detects traces of the drug. When the tox-screen result is positive, it is still not possible to know how affected the infant will be for two to three weeks, when the drug finally leaves the infant's body through excretory processes. There is one observable sign, however, that cues us that the drug exposure has been to cocaine: The baby does not wake to feed and takes less than one ounce of formula every three to four hours.

During the first two weeks of cocaine-exposed babies' lives, they mold into your body, snuggling up without fussiness or abnormal movements, and want to sleep most of the time. Your main reason for concern is likely to be their inability to take as much formula as they should for proper nutrition.

These babies' appearance will start to change between the seventh and fourteenth days of their lives. Body tone will begin to increase—muscles becoming more tense—and they may become slightly irritable, with a little more fussiness than you noticed earlier. With the increased muscle tone, you will see small muscle spasms or contractions—called myoclonic jerks—similar to what you may have experienced occasionally in a leg muscle, for example. These jerks are quite different from tremors, which go on for longer periods. (If we do see tremors in cocaine-exposed babies, we suspect that they have been exposed to some other drug in addition to cocaine.) Myoclonic jerks will occur most severely during deep sleep and will persist over several months. We have concluded that, even though monoclonic jerks appear to be painful, babies apparently are not bothered, except for being awakened by them. Feeding problems will also increase daily, with less and less formula being ingested. The time has clearly come for therapeutic handling.

Another common signal of cocaine exposure is frequent passing of gas, since these babies' gastric systems are affected. It may seem that the baby needs to excrete stool, but this is not so. The excessive gas is created by gastric contractions, not by normal passage of feces and gas through the intestines.

Feeding, of course, must be regular, even though the baby does not wake spontaneously. *Regularly*, in this case, means every three or four hours, for sure! During the first few days, one or two ounces per feeding may be the right amount. The amount must quickly and constantly increase so that within three weeks the baby is taking at least three ounces every three to four hours, and four ounces very soon after that. Any less is cause for worry.

Even when we get the baby up to two ounces, the greatest feeding problem has just begun. The baby will often become lethargic, hardly able to be wakened by your attentions, and when you try feeding, the baby will have no sucking power and may even try to fight the bottle. We speculate that a trigger in the brain somehow signals that a feeding is completed even before it has begun.

The manner of feeding is important. We've found that simply placing the nipple in the baby's mouth is not going to start the process. Here are other techniques we use:

- Support the baby's chin with your index finger.
- Curl the baby in a tight C-position.
- Use a two-ounce bottle rather than a larger one to get a faster flow of formula.
- Hold the baby away from your body to decrease the baby's comfort and make him more wakeful.
- Unswaddle the baby to increase wakefulness.
- Rub the baby's hands, feet, and top of the head, also to increase wakefulness.
- Pump the bottle back and forth in the baby's mouth four times, still with your index finger under the chin.
- Take the infant into a quiet room where concentration on feeding can be undisturbed.

At times other than feeding, we apply additional therapeutic-care techniques, such as swaddling, with a rolled thermal receiving blanket that helps mold and maintain the baby's body in a tight C-position as the baby lies on his or her side in a crib. This is the position the baby should be in most of the time because it helps control excessive body movements.

Although no drug support is needed for cocaine-affected babies, they must be closely monitored and carefully managed. Caregivers should use neonatal abstinence scoring (see Part IV) so that disturbances in the central nervous system (as well as metabolic, vasomotor, respiratory, and gastrointestinal disturbances) can be detected. The baby will begin to thrive if he or she has a highly consistent schedule of feeding and weighing, and if there is gradual daily introduction of stimuli.

Because this type of infant does not wake often to suckle and tends not to have normal weight gain, the schedule and conditions for feeding must be strict. Feeding the baby every three or four hours is a must. More frequent feedings are not advisable because they require too much of the infant's already diminished energy supply. If the feeding technique suggested earlier for encouraging sucking behavior does not work, your pediatrician may recommend a hypercaloric formula. This may be used long enough to achieve a suitable weight gain or until the infant can suckle normally and return to the usual formula.

While a strict feeding schedule is important, so are the conditions for feeding. It's best to set aside about forty-five minutes for each feeding, and be sure that you and the baby are in a calm and quiet place, where you are unlikely to be distracted or interrupted. By whatever means necessary, it is essential to make sure the cocaine-exposed baby is not allowed to deteriorate because of an inadequate diet. Because this baby is so much in need of nutrition, never dilute the infant's formula or give the baby water, unless your doctor has recommended that you do so. Otherwise, giving the baby water can be dangerous.

A strict feeding schedule may not relieve all gastric discomfort, because the return to normal function takes months. For the first six months—or even the first twelve—the child may have frequent gas and constipation. To relieve gastric distress, burp the baby well after each feeding. With gradual increase in muscle tone, the baby will overcome these symptoms.

We want to note the importance of faithfully continuing all the therapeutic-care techniques we have just explained. Stopping them too soon may cause the baby to revert to an earlier, less healthy stage. Anyone providing care for a cocaine-exposed child will see the benefits of controlled conditions, organized environments, and predictable routines.

We mentioned that reduction of environmental stimuli will be necessary if the cocaine-exposed infant becomes irritable. Finding the right balance of stimuli can be complicated. While we don't propose a rigid schedule for amount and kind of stimuli, we suggest below the major kinds of stimuli, each to be reduced and then reintroduced in lesser intensity over a period of days. The most important element is the caregiver's observations of the effects of each of these stimuli as they reenter the infant's environment:

- bright light
- music
- loud sounds, including talking
- face-to-face contact
- frequent handling
- strong smells
- high-energy visitors
- riding in a car
- crowds

None of these stimuli is inherently damaging to an infant, but the cocaine-exposed infant is likely to need carefully monitored dosages of each, just as amounts of formula consumption need to be carefully monitored.

Note: These same therapeutic care techniques can be used with infants whose exposure was to hallucinogens or inhalants.

Tammy: A Cocaine-Affected Baby

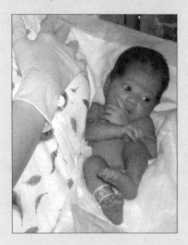

When Tammy came to us from a nearby local hospital, she was twelve hours old—born six weeks early, with prenatal exposure to cocaine. Nurses at the hospital reported that she was doing quite well, but when she arrived at the center, we noted that her color was not quite right and that her temperature was unstable.

We could see right away that she was having some trouble nippling from a bottle and that she needed a hypercaloric formula. She had no fatty tissue and was small for her gestational age—a result of the mother's poor nutrition during her pregnancy. Nevertheless, she was a beautiful baby. Often, when she was in deep sleep in a caregiver's arms or in her crib, she had myoclonic jerks in one of her extremities.

Over the next few days, nurses gave a great deal of encouragement to increase her sucking ability: chin-and-cheek support and concentrated therapeutic techniques. She needed frequent stimulation to increase her alertness, such as rubbing of her head, feet, and hands. Because she—like other cocaine-affected babies—was at high risk for failure to thrive, we monitored her weight closely.

When it was time for Tammy to leave the center, we stressed the importance of someone continuing these same techniques in the home. Unfortunately, the foster mother whom the caseworker chose was not willing to learn the appropriate feeding techniques or keep in touch with us about Tammy's progress. After three weeks with this caregiver, we found that Tammy had not gained the hoped-for weight, and she was being fed every two hours rather than every three or four. (Since each feeding burns calories and therefore retards the necessary weight gain, feedings need to be less frequent.) The caregiver expressed frustration to the caseworker, after the fifth week, that the baby was irritable, not eating the amounts she should, and therefore not gaining the appropriate two pounds a month. Experienced as she was as a foster mother, it was difficult for her to understand the importance of the special techniques needed to feed a cocaine-affected baby. She seemed not to grasp the fact that in-utero cocaine exposure definitely inhibits an infant's ability to eat. Otherwise, this caregiver provided the right environment for such a baby: a low-stimulus home and several necessary therapeutic-handling techniques.

Six months later, the baby was at a point where she was gaining weight and doing well. The caregiver now acknowledges that she wanted to do everything her own way and that she did not understand at first how to care for a baby with cocaine exposure. The caregiver is now doing well in controlling stimuli and Tammy may, by the time she is two or three years old, be able to manage her responses to stimuli.

Amphetamines and Methamphetamines (Stimulants)

The infant born to a mother who has used either amphetamines (taken orally) or methamphetamines (smoked) will, at first, appear to be perfectly healthy. The caregiver may even say at first this is a "good" baby, meaning that he or she sleeps a lot, seems to have no distress, and is soft and cuddly. What the caregiver cannot yet tell is that the drug stays in the infant's body for one to two weeks and has a generally depressive effect. That effect manifests as almost continuous sleeping and lack of need to feed. In such a baby, "good" really means lethargic—not at all a good sign. The tone of the whole body is low: the arms, legs, and head are floppy, much like the floppiness of a rag doll.

Signs of withdrawal from the drug usually appear no earlier than the seventh day of the amphetamine-exposed baby's life. Among the first signs are flickers of higher tone—muscles that appear slightly more tense, for example, when arching the back. Others include slight irritability, some improvement in sucking power, and ability to produce stool. After about two weeks, these signs will increase in intensity, signaling that the drug has for the most part left the system.

Although no pharmacological support is necessary for this type of drug exposure, close monitoring and careful management are essential. Neonatal abstinence scoring (see Part IV) is a must. This is the caregivers' ratings of disturbances in the central nervous system; metabolic, vasomotor, and respiratory disturbances; and gastrointestinal disturbances. Also, the caregiver must provide highly consistent scheduling—especially feeding and weighing—and therapeutic management—including gradual daily introduction of stimuli.

Because this type of infant does not wake often to suckle and tends not to have normal weight gain, the schedule and conditions for feeding must be strict. A bottle only every three or four hours is the goal. More frequent feedings are not advisable because they require too much of the infant's already diminished energy supply. If the feeding technique for encouraging sucking behavior (suggested for the cocaine-affected baby) does not work, your pediatrician may recommend that you use a hypercaloric formula long enough to achieve a suitable weight gain or until the infant can suckle normally and return to the usual formula.

While a strict feeding schedule is important, so are the conditions for feeding. It's best to set aside about forty-five minutes for each feeding, and be sure that you and the baby are in a calm and quiet place, where you are unlikely to be distracted or interrupted.

We stress that, by whatever means necessary, it is essential to make sure the amphetamine-exposed baby is not allowed to wither because of an inadequate diet. To thrive, he or she must eat. Making that happen is a primary responsibility.

Even as the feeding schedule is maintained, gastric discomfort may increase. The baby's digestive tract, having been affected by the drug exposure, takes considerable time to become normal. Therefore, for the first six months—or even the first twelve—the child may pass gas frequently and may have constipation. It helps to burp the baby well after each feeding to relieve any gastric distress. Then, as the baby's body gradually advances to a higher tone, the cause of the discomfort will disappear.

Higher tone, desirable as it is in the long run, needs to be controlled in the early weeks by using the C-position. Swaddled, the baby needs to be kept in this position at all times, whether lying down or in your arms.

These therapeutic techniques, faithfully applied during the infant's first months of life, will do much to assure normal development. However, stopping them too soon may cause setbacks. Any future caregivers, then, should be advised that amphetamine-exposed children need much the same tightly controlled conditions that you provided in infancy. The children benefit from organized environments, with clearly recognizable routines, as their bodies slowly become capable of handling the stresses of more relaxed environments.

Jared: An Amphetamine-Affected Baby

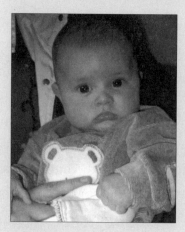

Hospital staff thought Jared was doing fine and could go to his grandmother's home or to foster care. He seemed to show no effects of prenatal amphetamine exposure. A case-worker was uneasy with this conclusion, however, and referred the baby to us.

Our examination showed him to be pink and cuddly but

with low muscle tone and a lethargic appearance. The effects of amphetamines, still in his body, were obvious to us. He had little or no suck and had to be encouraged to take enough formula. For a week, we had to gavage feed him (that is through a naso-gastric tube), using a hypercaloric formula.

When the mother and father visited after the first week, they made sincere efforts to feed Jared with a bottle, without success. He slept through their visits. We explained the cause: lack of muscle tone attributable to amphetamines still in his system. Gradually, normal tone would return, though not in all parts of the body at the same time. Only then would he be able to take enough formula through a nipple on a bottle to gain weight.

Use of the hypercaloric formula continued for a month, both because he weighed only four pounds, six ounces at birth and because of his lethargy. We needed to give more than the normal number of calories to make up for his nutritional deprivation before he was born.

Parental visits during this period were sporadic and involved little nurturing behavior. The father said little; the mother easily became irritated. According to our observations, their ability to be suitable parents was in question; nevertheless, the caseworker decided to send Jared home to be with the mother and father, who were living with the maternal grandmother. That arrangement lasted for one week, until we received emergency calls to go to the house and get the baby into a safe environment. Jared then went to his paternal grandmother, where he fared well.

Heroin and Methadone (Opiates)

Within twenty-four to forty-eight hours after birth, the heroin- or methadone-exposed baby shows symptoms of withdrawal: frantic movement, a high-pitched cry (we call it a cat cry), tremors, inability to sleep or suck a bottle, fast breathing, and frequent and loose stools. These symptoms are likely to be more severe in methadone-exposed babies than in those heroin-exposed; for that reason, post-birth treatment for methadone babies usually includes prescribed narcotic drugs.

Whether or not to prescribe drugs is determined during these babies' first two weeks of life. We monitor their symptoms closely to know whether our usual techniques need to be supplemented by medication. If so, a physician prescribes the drugs and a clinic like ours or a hospital administers the drugs. One of the dangers inherent in the use of a prescribed narcotic drug is overdose, which could result in depressing or stopping the infant's ability to breathe. Therefore, constant monitoring of the drug's effects is essential.

With or without the use of a prescribed narcotic drug, therapeutic-handling techniques are essential. The usual C-position for both holding and sleeping is especially important. It may be necessary to try various holding positions of the tightly swaddled baby—held close, held away from the caregiver's body, vertical rocking, or slow and rhythmic sideways swaying—for only a few seconds to determine which is best. Making a shushing sound, but not speaking directly into the baby's face, is also comforting to such a frantic baby.

Babies exposed to an opiate such as heroin or methadone

also need several of the same therapeutic-care techniques as those whose prenatal exposure was to stimulants, such as cocaine. And these same techniques can be used for infants whose exposure was to hallucinogens or inhalants.

A very important technique is swaddling: the rolled cotton-thermal receiving blanket helping to mold and maintain the baby's body in a tight C-position as the baby lies on his or her side in a crib. Because the swaddled C-position helps control excessive body movements, the baby should be in this position most of the time.

Reducing environmental stimuli also benefits the opiate-exposed infant. Each stimulus can be reduced and then reintroduced in lesser intensity over a period of days: bright light; music; loud sounds, including talking; face-to-face contact; frequent handling; strong smells; and high-energy caregivers. While none of these stimuli is necessarily damaging, the heroin- or methadone-exposed infant takes comfort in carefully controlled exposure to these stimuli.

Because of all their disorganized activity, heroin- or methadone-exposed babies use a lot of energy and therefore need a diet high in calories and frequent feedings—every three instead of every four hours. Without them, weight loss is almost a certainty. Aggravating the feeding problem is a disorganized suck—inability to grasp onto the nipple compared to what we usually see in normal infants—or maybe a suck that is excessively strong, which can cause choking.

Other problems may include rapid breathing, sweating, gas, and continued inability to sleep. A baby with so many problems is more than a handful. It's a difficult job to keep trying various ways of calming and nourishing the infant, but these children are in the power of a substance that produces frantic behaviors. Dealing with these infants takes an informed and versatile caregiver, and the rewards are great when we help gradually gain control of their bodies and eat properly.

The caregiver for a baby exposed to heroin or methadone has a difficult and intense job. It can help to stop and think:

- Am I able to maintain or regain my calm?
- Am I organized in my caregiving techniques?
- Do I maintain a schedule that includes carefully recorded results of my observations?
- Am I able to maintain an energy level that helps me to be vigilant and consistent with my therapeutic-handling techniques?
- Am I part of a community of caregivers that can help me sustain my commitment to dealing properly with this infant?
- Do I have ways to learn and try new techniques to supplement or replace those I am using?

Doing the right thing for these babies is not easy. It takes extraordinary effort to be a successful giver of care for them. It also requires detective work to watch for danger signs. Some of the actions listed below are for the caregiver, while others require a physician or medical assistant.

DANGER SIGNS	HOSPITAL ACTIONS
Large number of stools or stools turning to water (both indicate internal withdrawals). Also note: Stools may be explosive, acidic, and may contain blood. They will burn buttocks rapidly and produce open wounds.	1. Act fast. 2. Consider use of morphine (with physician's prescription) to rest the gut. 3. If morphine does not help, put baby on Pedialite (in place of formula) for twenty-four hours and then an easily digestible formula such as Nutramigen or Alimentum. Also note: Closely monitor the effects of these formulas because they may not produce adequate weight gain. Consult with a physician to determine proper caloric content of formula.
Cat cry, often associated with frantic behavior (called *cat cry* because it is high-pitched and unlike any other infant cry) and heard during first two weeks of withdrawal; also can be associated with frequent, burning stools.	1. Meet baby's needs immediately upon awakening, to avoid baby getting out of control. 2. Provide experienced caregiver — not a high-energy person. 3. Use neonatal abstinence scoring as a guide, but let the baby be the principal source of information about how to proceed with treatment.

Josie: A Heroin-Affected Baby

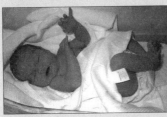

Josie is a beautiful blonde baby girl who recently "graduated" from our center's program. Both of her parents are addicted to heroin, a habit that overwhelmed their desire to provide proper care and nurture for their beautiful baby.

Josie was four days old when she came to the center from a local hospital. In the early stage of withdrawal from heroin and methadone, she had moderate to severe tremors, a high-pitched cry, and explosive stools. She had already been placed

Drug Types, Specific Drugs, and Their Effects

on a fairly high dose of morphine (.70 milliliters every three hours, administered by mouth), and her neonatal abstinence score ranged from fourteen to eighteen. We immediately put her on a cardio-respiratory monitor because the morphine dose was so high, and we evaluated her to make sure she was stable.

One of our first observations noted her limited ability to take in formula—only one ounce without additional encouragement in the form of therapeutic handling. As the time neared for her morphine dose, she became frantic and resisted efforts to calm her down. Stools also became more explosive and consisted almost entirely of liquid. All these symptoms convinced us that her morphine dose was too low and that we needed to increase it rapidly.

Swaddling her after our assessment, we moved her into our low-stimulus room and increased her morphine dose to offer her more support and decrease the watery stools. Through the night, the nurse made every effort to keep Josie calm. The stools slowed, but didn't stop. Her nippling ability improved, doubling her hypercaloric formula intake. This greater amount of food was important because her frantic behavior and her efforts to control it were burning up calories, a process that would quickly lead to weight loss.

Her tremors continued over the next few days, and she required intensive therapeutic handling. Her high-pitched cat cry continued; her stools decreased but were still watery. We could see that we would have to increase the morphine dose again. The result was that we finally did stabilize her—returning stools to a safe consistency, increasing her formula intake, and requiring less intensive therapeutic handling. Her cry, however, continued to have the catlike quality, and she had difficulty sleeping.

In these early days, Josie's mother and father came frequently to see her and started learning therapeutic-handling techniques. They had great difficulty, however, with Josie's frantic behavior; they asked earnestly and often how to quiet her. However, their eager presence would overstimulate the baby. During the process of decreasing her morphine dose, the baby became more irritable. This led to less frequent parental visits of shorter duration; the emotional strain on them was all too evident.

By the fourth week, we had reduced the morphine dosage by half. Josie was doing much better, though she still required considerable therapeutic support. She responded to swaddling and cuddling provided by caregivers, who now seldom included the parents. Their visits were down to about a half-hour once a week, and their behavior was changing: they smelled of alcohol, the mother held the baby only for brief periods, the father smiled less and held the baby hardly at all. Ironically, as the baby continued to thrive and smiled occasionally, showing every sign of engaging with caregivers, the parents abandoned her, apparently having succumbed entirely to heroin. This is the heartbreaking pattern we often see.

The picture is not entirely bleak, however. Relatives came forward when they heard about Josie. They volunteered to come to the center to learn care techniques. When they appeared, they were so excited that they took in little of what we told them. We decided to delay slightly Josie's departure with them. Two days later, after they had calmed themselves enough to hear and understand our instructions, they showed every sign that they could be wonderful caregivers, aware that the quality of their care would directly determine whether Josie would continue to progress. We, of course, wanted her to have the best possible chance of growing healthily, as, indeed, she has done with these foster parents.

Psychotropics (Anti-psychotic Prescription Drugs)

The effects on infants of prenatal exposure to psychotropic drugs are difficult to detect at birth. The babies initially seem normal, but have difficulty with feeding, and need a strictly observed schedule. A significant difference in the psychotropic-exposed baby, however, is sensitivity to stimuli. Being held in most of the positions a caregiver can think of worsens the symptoms, as do most environmental stimuli, including the nipple on the formula bottle.

For about the first three weeks of the child's life, the infant will seem normal, sleeping and eating as you would expect a newborn to do and responding to mild stimuli in accustomed ways. But then the changes accelerate rapidly—changes associated with the drug leaving the baby's system. Suckling becomes a struggle, with screaming and movements aimed at pushing the nipple out of the mouth. Light and sound of even the slightest intensity also trigger frantic movements, which, in turn, can easily trigger a feeling of desperation in any but the most experienced and resourceful caregiver.

The greatest danger to the well-being of such an infant—as it is with amphetamine-exposed infants—is failure to gain weight. Consequently, the caregiver's priority is to give an adequate amount of formula to the baby. How to do this when he or she consistently fights the nipple? The solution is to engage in a kind of subtle swaying. Alone with the baby and concentrating fully on the baby's responses, you may try many different holding positions, always searching for the one that has the greatest soothing effect: C-position, immobility, holding the infant away from you, vertical rock, head-to-toe movement, and clapping. By trying each of these—and variations on them—you will, we expect, eventually discover a position that reduces the hypersensitivity, even if it is just for a few seconds. Your victories may be small ones when the infant is in this delicate phase, but they are very important.

As a result of these small victories, the infant will likely consume less liquid than he or she really needs, so a period of using hypercaloric formula (as prescribed by your pediatrician) may well be necessary. Don't hesitate to describe the feeding difficulty to your doctor and show your records of feeding times and amounts. Then leave it to the doctor's judgment as to whether a formula change is called for.

Because you will become highly attuned to the baby's hypersensitivity to all stimuli, you may be tempted to use only a night-light and reduce sounds. However, it is best, after an initial period of greatly reduced stimuli, to daily introduce stimuli by very small increments. You might gradually use your voice (talking and singing) a little more often and a little more loudly as you provide care. The aim, of course, is to find the tolerance level of the child to normal kinds of sensory stimuli—a process that differs for each child and that you can monitor only by being extremely observant of the baby's reactions. If the response to any of these stimuli seems too great to you, cut the stimulus by half and offer that half the next day. You need to become the mediator between a distressed nervous system and the buzzing world of crowds, movement, sound, and light that this nervous system is going to have to adapt to.

Alcohol Exposure

Alcohol exposure is hard to trace and diagnose; therefore, being able to offer support to these infants is very difficult and elusive. This is unfortunate because alcohol exposure is the most damaging drug, with irreversible effects on the child and destructive effects on the family.

A CAREGIVER'S CONTINUING RESPONSIBILITIES

Early intervention and good care for the drug-exposed infant does a lot to permit later normal development. However, developmental problems do not end with infancy. While each baby differs, the effects of intrauterine drug exposure for many can be long-lasting and may lead to a child's being misdiagnosed as having attention deficit hyperactivity disorder (ADHD). The symptoms of the two conditions may be very similar, but the appropriate treatments are very different. ADHD is often treated with drugs that are similar to the very drugs that set off your baby's symptoms. Such treatment, as you can readily guess, would be a grave mistake. You must do everything you can to alert other caregivers, day-care workers, and teachers to this child's need for controlled exposure to stimuli, not more medications.

As the child matures, various negative behaviors—screaming, not sitting still at appropriate times, or talking back—may occur, perhaps with greater frequency or intensity than in other immature children. An adult seeing these behaviors may be quick to blame them on the prenatal drug exposure. A more useful response is to examine the child's present environment. Is environmental stimuli at a level the child can tolerate? Have reductions of stimuli been consistent? Has the caregiver carefully observed and recorded the situations that seem to trigger the child's more uncontrolled responses? Is there a quiet, nonstimulating place in the environment where the overacting child can go to "shut down?" Does every adult who comes into contact with the child understand and practice the necessary stimuli-limiting disciplines? Until the answer to all these questions is "yes," it is a mistake to blame either the misbehaving child or the prenatal drug exposure as the cause of the problem.

This is not to say, however, that the type of prenatal drug exposure is irrelevant to later caregiving procedures. If the exposure was to heroin or methadone, maintaining a low-stimulus environment will be especially critical; this includes a caregiver whose temperament is low-key or low-energy. And if the situation involves day care, the adults in charge must have strong parenting skills and be responsible for only a small number of children. They must also be trained in therapeutic handling, as we have described it here, including a strict feeding schedule if the child is still in infancy.

If the exposure was to cocaine, methamphetamines, or amphetamines, a special care situation is also needed, though it may be one in which control of environmental stimuli can be somewhat less strict. A child with this kind of exposure can fare well with a caregiver who has strong child-care skills and fairly low personal energies. However, feeding during infancy remains a high priority: use of the special feeding techniques we have described, completion of each feeding, and observance of a regular feeding schedule are necessary.

When the child enters more formal schooling, he or she needs an advocate—a parent or caregiver who can explain to teachers what the child needs. These requirements include:

- Classroom management that features clear boundaries, discipline, and routine.
- Awareness of signs or signals of overstimulation, such as growing anxiousness, hyperactivity, or irritability.

Without seeming to tell the teacher how to teach, the caregiver can point out the need for early intervention, before the overstimulation gets out of hand. A special place where the child goes to "shut down" can be a special chair. For one little boy we know, it was a refrigerator box on the floor. When the teacher sees signs of overstimulation, he or she can take the child firmly by the hand to the special place, making it clear that this is not a punishment; it's just a need for some quiet time. Soon, the child will go there without an adult's guidance.

If both teachers and home caregivers react to warning signs consistently, these overstimulated children will soon learn to recognize the signals on their own. They'll know when they need to pull back, go to their room, or just sit down for a while. As they grow older, caregivers can talk with them about the things that give them trouble, letting them know that they always have choices for the things they can't handle.

And you'll probably find that there will always be things your child can't handle. One child, after many years, still has trouble looking out the side window of the car; all that scenery flashing by is too stimulating. She's learned to focus her vision ahead. When she was little, she used to stand at the door and peek around when there were a lot of people in a room; she was uncomfortable with crowds and always stayed on the fringes. Crowds, stores, fluorescent lights, people with high-energy levels: some things will always be hard. But with a little help and understanding, most kids can find a way through or around them.

You can expect, too, to hit some bumps in the road as drug-exposed children grow. We've found that there tend to be some predictably difficult times when it may seem that your child is going backward. These tend to happen at around six months, two years, the beginning of school, and again at adolescence. All of these are times of transition, and it usually takes these children a little longer to adjust to new situations.

Good parenting for any child is not easy. For those who started life with the handicap of drug exposure, parenting involves continuous vigilance about environmental conditions and special intervention efforts. The reward for this special care can be a loving, productive, and happy adult.

IV

Record Keeping

You have seen us refer several times to the Finnegan tool (or neonatal abstinence scoring). In noting the importance of daily records for infant behavior, we have, we hope, impressed you with the nurselike behavior that is essential during drug-exposed babies' first weeks and months of life. Nurses keep meticulous records in order to monitor the signs of health or dysfunction in each patient; only then can they and physicians know the patterns of signs that suggest the most appropriate treatment.

While most caregivers are not and don't have to be nurses, they do need to watch for patterns. Is the baby gaining weight steadily? Is muscle tone changing noticeably? Is the cry changing in pitch and intensity? Are tremors or myoclonic jerks persisting or changing in frequency? There are so many signs and symptoms like these to be monitored that no caregiver's memory can recall them over a period of weeks. And even with a stunning memory for such facts, you cannot persuade a pediatrician of what you have observed without a written record to show.

If you have never kept a daily chart of infant behavior, your first attempts may seem an intrusion on your time. Appropriately, you may be concentrating so much on the baby that you will forget or resent the extra time it takes to write numbers and words on a sheet of paper. However, once you start doing it, you will find it a natural part of your care routine and a great help to you in understanding your infant.

Dr. Loretta Finnegan, from the University of Chicago, is a researcher on behavior of drug-exposed infants. She has developed a means of keeping efficient track of vital signs in these babies. Called the Finnegan Tool, it gives definitions of behavior and a numerical scoring system that helps you see patterns of behavior—patterns related to the effectiveness of care. We have adapted the Finnegan Tool for use twenty-four hours a day at the center; which we call the Neonatal Abstinence Scoring System (in other words, our method of keeping track of signs of drug withdrawal in newborns and young children).

The scoring system has three main categories: central nervous system (CNS) disturbances; metabolic, vasomotor, respiratory disturbances; and gastrointestinal disturbances. Each of these categories is described by observable signs or symptoms, and each has an assigned number or score. Every time you use the tool, you will determine if the infant is displaying a sign or symptom, and if he or she does, you will write the corresponding number within a box. (For example, if you observe that the infant often has a high-pitched cry, you will write 2 in a box under observation #.) The entire scoring sheet appears in the appendix in a form that you may copy. Following is an excerpt to show you how it looks:

system	signs & symptoms	score	observation # (by hours of day) 00 01 02 03 04 05 06 07 08 09
CNS	excessive high-pitched (or other) cry	2	
	continuous high-pitched cry	3	
	sleeps less than one hour after feeding	3	

The normal interval for scoring is every three hours, though, if the total score is higher than 8, scoring should occur every two hours. When scores are high at three successive scoring intervals—while you are using the recommended therapeutic-care techniques—the need for medication is likely. (Other indicators are an average greater than 8 on three consecutive scorings; a score greater than 12 on two consecutive scorings; or an average greater than 12 on two consecutive scorings.)

Besides the sheet on which you record scores, you will need a thermometer, a watch or clock with a second hand, and of course, your own sharp eyes for noticing the many important signs.

Now, you need to know what to look for. Following you will find explanations and instructions for each of the signs and symptoms:

CENTRAL NERVOUS SYSTEM DISTURBANCES
Crying

Excessive high-pitched crying (perhaps to the point of shrillness) continuous or intermittent for *up to five* minutes in spite of attempts to comfort.

Continuous high-pitched crying for *greater than five* minutes in spite of attempts to comfort.

*Note: If infant cries before feeding and stops when fed, this is **not** excessive or continuous crying.*

Sleep

Score should be for longest sleep interval within entire two- or three-hour scoring period, not when infant has been disturbed for whatever reason.

Score only one of the three boxes pertaining to sleep (that is when scored for less than two hours, don't also score for less than three hours).

Score only when infant wakes on his or her own. (For example if infant sleeps for seventy minutes, wakes for thirty minutes, and sleeps again for seventy minutes, score as less than two hours during interval because longest sleep period was less than two hours. If infant wakes only briefly, it is not counted as a sleep interruption.)

Moro Reflex

[DEFINITION: When infant is lifted slightly off mattress by wrists to a semi-sitting position and is allowed to fall back onto mattress, he or she straightens arms, moves them out at the elbows into a C-shape, and returns arms to chest in a flexion, or resting position. Extension of knees and hip joints, followed by flexion, may also occur. Slight jitteriness in the form of a tremor and crying may also occur.] Score only one of the following categories:

Score as **hyperactive** (2) when infant has pronounced jitteriness of hands during reflex.

Score as **hypersensitive** (3) when infant has both jitteriness and repetitive jerking of wrist or ankle.

Tremors

[DEFINITION: Involuntary, rhythmical movements of a limb or other part of body; some tremor during sleep is normal and not scorable in this category.] Score only one of the following categories:

Mild disturbed (score of 1) when infant has observable tremors of **hands or feet** while being handled, whether asleep or awake.

Moderate-severe disturbed (score of 2) when infant has tremors of **arms and/or legs** while being handled (with or without involvement of hands or feet).

Mild undisturbed (score of 3) when infant has tremors of **hands or feet** while **not** being handled.

Moderate-severe undisturbed (score of 4) when infant has tremors of **arms or legs** while **not** being handled.

Note: An infant who has mild tremors while undisturbed (score of 3) is likely to have moderate-severe tremors while disturbed (score of 2); use the higher score in such a case.

Increased Muscle Tone

[DEFINITION OF TONE: Muscles recoil or spring back to original position when stretched.]

Score only when infant is awake and calm by slowly pulling infant into sitting position or by extending arms and legs; observe whether head lags and infant remains rigid or whether arms and legs flex tightly and resist gentle extension (both signs of increased muscle tone, score of 2).

Excoriation

[DEFINITION: Breakdown of skin resulting from rubbing against a flat surface.] Score only when excoriation occurs in areas other than diaper, such as, chin, knees, elbows, toes, and fingers.

Myoclonic Jerks

[DEFINITION: Involuntary, quick and jerky (short in duration) muscle spasms, occurring singly or in succession in face or extremities.] Score separately from tremors, which are quivering and rhythmical, not jerky.

Convulsions/Seizures

[DEFINITION: Generalized myoclonic jerks involving more than one extremity, either subtly or more obviously—as in rapid eye movement, chewing, rowing of arms, bicycling of legs, back arching, or fist clenching.] Score when any of these generalized jerks occur.

Note: When caregiver notes such signs, he or she should touch or flex the extremity; if it is a seizure, intervention will have no effect.

METABOLIC, VASOMOTOR, AND RESPIRATORY DISTURBANCES

Sweating

Score if infant's forehead, upper lip, or back of neck feels wet.

Note: If overheating from swaddling seems to be causing sweating, do not score this category.

Fever

Score either of these categories:

Score as (1) if infant's temperature is between 99 and 101 degrees Fahrenheit.

Score as (2) if infant's temperature is higher than 101 degrees Fahrenheit.

Note: Take infant's temperature with glass thermometer held for at least three minutes under infant's armpit.

Frequent Yawning

Score when infant yawns more than three times during observation period.

Mottling

[DEFINITION: Discoloration of skin resembling marbling, typically on chest, trunk, arms, or legs.] Score when mottling is visible.

Note: Do not score when mottling occurs because of chilling after bath or when infant has been left uncovered for an extended period.

Nasal Stuffiness

Score when mucous partially blocks infant's nostrils (whether or not you can see it) and breathing is noisy.

Sneezing

Score when infant sneezes more than three times during observation period.

Nasal Flaring

[DEFINITION: Outward spreading of nostrils during breathing.] Score when flaring is present.

Respiratory Rate

Score when rate of in-and-out breaths is greater than sixty per minute.

Note: Count each in-and-out breath as one, and count for a full minute, while infant is calm. Also, note whether infant sucks in chest wall, above or around rib cage (called retractions), producing labored breathing.

GASTROINTESTINAL DISTURBANCES
Frantic or Disorganized Suck

Score as (3) when infant's suck is disorganized (that is, unable to latch on to nipple or close mouth), or frantic (that is, shaking head, mouthing nipple, or dribbling).

Excessive Sucking

Score as (1) when infant grasps nipple so strongly that caregiver must break seal to release, or when infant roots more than three times to suck on pacifier or fist.

Flatus (Gas)

Score as (1) when gas occurs.

Poor Feeding

Score if infant has excessive sucking before feeding, infrequently sucks during feeding, or has uncoordinated suck.

Note: If infant sucks so as to consume less than minimum intake during specified time (usually thirty to forty-five minutes), consider this poor feeding.

Regurgitation

[DEFINITION: Non-projectile vomiting of gastric contents during or after feeding and not associated with burping.] Score if infant has two or more regurgitation episodes during feeding or regurgitates less than 1/4 oz. between feedings.

Projectile Vomiting

[DEFINITION: Forceful ejection of stomach contents during or after feeding.] Score whenever infant vomits forcefully.

Loose Stools

[DEFINITION: Bowel movement (stool) appears curdy, seedy, or runny, without a water ring and semiliquid or liquid.] Score when infant's stool has any of these qualities.

Water-Ring Stools

[DEFINITION: Stool is soft with a water ring surrounding it.]

Watery Stools

[DEFINITION: Stool has little substance.]

If all these explanations of signs and symptoms and the instructions for scoring them seem complicated, we urge you to be patient. After a few days of working with a drug-exposed baby and keeping track of what you observe, you are likely to find the process easier and a normal part of the care you provide. And when you show your chart to your pediatrician, you will be further gratified by how helpful this information is in teaming with the doctor to care for your infant.

NEONATAL ABSTINENCE SCORING SYSTEM

Date: _____

			Time:										
Central Nervous System Disturbances	Excessive High Pitched (or other) Cry	2											
	Continuous High Pitched (or other) Cry	3											
	Sleeps < 1 Hour After Feeding	3											
	Sleeps < 2 Hours After Feeding	2											
	Sleeps < 3 Hours After Feeding	1											
	Hyperactive Moro Reflex	2											
	Hypersensitivity	3											
	Markedly Hyperactive Moro Reflex	3											
	Mild Tremors Disturbed	1											
	Moderate-Severe Tremors Disturbed	2											
	Mild Tremors Undisturbed	3											
	Moderate-Severe Tremors Undisturbed	4											
	Increased Muscle Tone	2											
	Excoriation (specify area)	1											
	Monoclonic Jerks	3											
	Convulsions/Seizures	5											
Metabolic, Vasomotor Respiratory Disturbances	Sweating	1											
	Fever > 99-101 (37.3C to 38.3C)	1											
	Fever > 101 (38.4C or higher)	2											
	Frequent Yawning (>3-4/interval)	1											
	Mottling	1											
	Nasal Stuffiness	1											
	Sneezing (>3-4 times/interval)	1											
	Nasal Flaring	2											
	Respiratory Rate > 60/minute	1											
Gastro-Intestinal Disturbances	Disorganized Suck	3											
	Excessive Sucking	1											
	Flatus	1											
	Poor Feeding	2											
	Regurgitation	2											
	Projectile Vomiting	3											
	Loose Stools	2											
	Water Ring Stools	2											
	Watery Stools	3											
	TOTAL SCORE												
	INITIALS OF SCORER												

V

Dealing with Drug-Dependent Mothers

For most people who have had little direct experience with drug-affected infants, the range of types of their mothers comes as a surprise. We have dealt with hundreds of them: women from every walk of life, ethnic and cultural background, and socioeconomic level. Some have borne several children; some have careers in professional fields; some have husbands and otherwise intact families; some are homeless and destitute.

There is no generalization to be made, it seems, about who the biological mothers of drug-affected babies are. The reality of our care center has broken all the stereotypes of drug-affected children and their families. Most of the families are suburban and middle class. Eighty percent are Caucasian. Most are twenty-five to thirty-five years of age. We've found that drug addiction crosses all racial and economic groups.

It is hard not to feel sadness for these mothers—sadness that their drug-dependence is causing them to suffer so much at a time when most women are finding joy in motherhood. For many of them, their pregnancies did not seem real until the babies were born. After they give birth, we see them feeling guilt and grief about their babies' conditions, as well as remorse and embarrassment about their addictions. It's hard to see them hurting. We know they fear that their drug-exposed infants may face a greater risk of being drug abusers later on in life, or have a predisposition for addiction.

We have seen as many as eight babies from one mother. This is not carelessness. This is a testament to the power of addiction. The guilt of addicted mothers is horrendous to watch. They know how withdrawal feels and they know that they have caused their babies to suffer. The mothers are children too, who need our help and protection. By keeping the babies medically safe, we are helping the mothers, too.

While we feel for the mothers, our main focus is on guiding the babies through the intense headaches, chills, stomach cramps, tremors, and gastric distress—the same symptoms that an adult suffers during withdrawal. If the mothers say they want to parent their children, we welcome them, and we are firm with them. We all must focus on the best interests of the babies.

GENERALIZATIONS THAT MAY APPLY TO DRUG-ABUSING MOTHERS:
- They have only a small chance of kicking the habit and staying drug-free.
- They will feel guilt and embarrassment about not being able to perform well as mothers.
- They may lie about their behavior out of a sense of shame.
- They may exhibit dangerous behavior, especially when agitated.

- Some formerly drug-abusing mothers are trainable in maternal skills.
- Drug-addicted mothers should not breast-feed their babies.

We elaborate below on each of these observations so that you may apply them in your own situation, whether it be foster care or an extended family.

Chances of Staying Drug-Free

For a woman with a long history of drug use, the likelihood of staying drug-free after the baby's birth is remote. Statistically, there is a ninety-seven percent overall chance of her returning to old habits; a mother's dependency usually overcomes whatever determination to quit she may have felt. If she continues to abuse drugs, she will not be able to provide for her baby in anymore than minimal ways. For a woman who may have been legally required to enter an inpatient treatment center as a condition of caring for her child, no less than a full year of such treatment is likely to give her a chance of staying drug-free.

Feelings of Guilt and Embarrassment

Seldom does a drug-addicted mother feel good about what she has done to her baby or about her inability to provide proper mothering. She may not admit that inability to anyone else; she may seem belligerent as a way to cover her guilt and embarrassment.

Caregivers, therefore, need to learn how to combine sympathy with firmness. They may hear stories from a mother that, for example, members of her family are responsible for her drug use. In contrast, members of her extended family may simply have become burned out after years of trying to support her and have distanced themselves from her. Facing their unwillingness to indulge her habit, she feels abandonment, desperation and deepened feelings of guilt, which lead her to turn that guilt back on the family, as she accuses them of withholding food, housing, clothing, and medical assistance for the baby. Knowing that they must not involve themselves with pleas for money, family members can supply food, clothing, or medical care directly.

A principal reason for our adding social workers to our care-center staff was to assist in these very kinds of situations. Caregivers in other settings may find that they, too, need assistance from professionals such as social workers in order to try to prevent desperate family situations from spiraling out of control and harming the infant.

Lying about Behavior

Be aware that a mother who wants her baby and who is also using drugs is in a great deal of conflict. She may lie and use manipulative behavior to get what she wants.

In our experience, for example, a mother was required to make daily trips to a methadone clinic as a means for altering her heroin addiction. After those visits, she came to our center for a two- to three-hour visit with her baby. Often, as she sat holding him, she nodded off (a result partly of the methadone and certainly because of the low stimulation in the center environment). When a staff member tried to take the baby from her, she protested, "No, I wasn't asleep. I was just resting my eyes." It was a small lie, certainly, but it showed a mother's desire to care for her child. We had to be firm with her for the sake of the baby's safety.

Another mother had been abusing cocaine and, after her baby's birth, was legally required to take regular urine tox-screen tests to prove cocaine abstinence. Thin and highly energetic, she made infrequent visits to the center. Whenever the tox-screen results were positive, she argued that the results were wrong or that someone else's urine had been substituted for hers.

It may seem mean-spirited for caregivers to suspect mothers of manipulation. But it's better to understand the possible motives and ensure that the babies stay safe.

Dangerous Behavior

A mother who smells of cat urine may have been cooking and using methamphetamines. If so, she is extremely toxic and must not come near you or the baby you are caring for. In such a case, one must try to avoid any confrontational behavior that might further agitate the mother for fear that she will injure you or the baby.

Training in Maternal Skills

Many of the mothers can learn to become effective caregivers. For those who have never before given birth, the task is new, made all the more difficult to learn by the baby's frantic behavior. Even if they had children before their addiction to drugs, they have to relearn maternal skills, which have apparently been submerged or wiped out by the effects of drug use.

Mothers frequently come to the center and expect their babies to be awake and responsive when they enter the room. And they can feel terribly hurt or rejected when they feel their babies arch away from being held. In such cases, we explain that the baby is incapable of feeling hatred; it's just that the stimulation of human contact is so difficult for a drug-exposed baby. We begin teaching them the therapeutic-handling techniques to decrease the babies' discomforts. Later, when the baby has stabilized, the mothers become more involved in feedings.

We surround our mothers with services and explanations/demonstrations of every procedure from swaddling to bathing. Our aim is for a smooth and unthreatening transition from the mother's feelings of ineptness to her acceptance of consistent, careful handling. This most definitely includes learning to read the infant's signs and symptoms so that they are not misreading and therefore mis-responding. Above all, we aim to avoid or reduce the tendency to feel overwhelmed so that the mothers will be less tempted to seek out drugs again simply as a way of reducing frustration.

Urging against Breast-feeding

Mothers in treatment are required to submit to urinalysis only once a month. Such infrequent testing cannot document actual drug usage and therefore gives us no assurance that the mothers with babies at our center are within allowable limits. With the safety of the infants of primary importance, we decided not to allow breast-feeding at all.

We became sure of that decision through discussions with groups of mothers on methadone. For every group of ten mothers, we usually learned that three or four were breast-feeding. They reasoned that if they stopped, they would have irritable babies instead of ones who simply ate and slept all the time. One woman said that her daily dose of methadone was 119 milligrams and that she breast-fed only at night, "Because my baby sleeps better." (Medical literature of the early 1990s suggested breast-feeding was permissible only if the mother was on less than twenty-one milligrams of methadone per twenty-four-hour day.)

This case pales in comparison to another case of a mother who had begun to split her daily methadone dose with her baby! Fortunately, through intervention by a methadone-treatment counselor, the baby was admitted to our center, where we applied appropriate treatment for withdrawal. When we talked to this mother, she claimed that, soon after the baby's birth, hospital staff had strongly encouraged her to breast-feed, although, in her words, "It was not something I wanted to do." When the baby was one month old, her breast milk had dried up, and the baby became fussy and tremulous. That's when she began splitting her methadone dose to calm the infant.

The three-week-old baby of another methadone-treated, breast-feeding mother came to our center at the mother's request, even though she knew we do not allow breast-feeding. The baby was on .20 milliliters of morphine every three hours and needed our help. Having breast-fed immediately before entry to the center, the baby showed increasing signs of withdrawal within fifteen hours, and her neonatal abstinence scores were between twelve and fourteen every three hours. We increased the morphine dose, because the baby was no longer ingesting methadone, and gradually accomplished complete withdrawal, without any further breast-feeding.

When drug use is involved, the most important client is the baby. If we protect the baby from further damage by tainted breast milk, we also protect the mother from inflicting that damage, even though she usually does not intend to harm her baby. (See the most recent recommendations of the American Academy of Pediatrics later in the next section.)

We can summarize our experience with breast-feeding by drug-affected mothers by offering these recommendations:

- Do not encourage chemically dependent mothers to breast-feed unless you have a tracking program in place—one that assures that the mother is not still using a drug.
- Have the mother undergo drug testing at least weekly.
- Request that tests be for all drugs, including alcohol.
- Request a printout from the lab of all drug-test results.
- Consider a urinalysis test "dirty" if the mother does not show up for an appointed test.
- Remember that all mothers want to do what is right for their babies; their drug use overwhelms their knowledge that breast-feeding while still taking drugs is harmful.

VI

Conversations with Pediatricians and Conclusion

Caring for drug-affected infants often involves a pediatrician, whether the caregiver has private access or seeks it through some public agency. As the use of illicit drugs has increased, pediatricians are seeing more babies who are in withdrawal or who are still showing the effects of in utero drug use. How are they reacting to this problem, and where do they place it on a scale of danger to the long-term well-being of these children?

Because caregivers may want to hear the opinions of highly respected pediatricians with considerable experience in the area of drug-exposed infants, we offer excerpts from our conversations with three pediatricians from the Puget Sound region, who have worked extensively at our center.

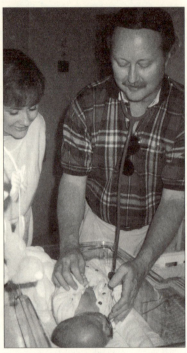

Dr. Peyton Gaunt, Medical Director and Staff Nurse, Debbie Will

DR. PEYTON GAUNT

Dr. Gaunt has been an attending pediatrician at the center from its earliest days. In mid-career at Valley Medical Center in Renton, Washington, he has a large private practice—one that includes babies and children from many economic and social backgrounds. He volunteers his time with us, both because he has special expertise in the medical problems resulting from maternal drug use, and because he thinks this huge problem requires small steps toward solution by anyone who wants to make a social contribution.

We see him and Dr. David Woodrum (a pediatrician and neonatologist from the University of Washington) at the center for part of one day every two weeks. He makes the rounds of all the babies in residence, examining them and checking treatment procedures (for example, establishing standing orders about feeding policies and administration of morphine) with our nurses. He is also on call for any emergencies that require a medical opinion.

Dr. Gaunt cites feeding difficulties as "one of the biggest problems with cocaine- and amphetamine-exposed babies."

They're at risk for getting inadequate calories. If they don't feed well, they don't grow well. We therefore have to do what might be described as therapeutic encouragement during feedings.

With drug-abusing mothers, Dr. Gaunt takes a patient attitude and avoids confrontation. All of his actions and suggestions are offered with the babies' best interests in mind. He believes that the mother needs to kick her drug habit if she has any hope of being the kind of mother her child needs. While he knows that the success rate for stopping drug use is historically low, he takes some comfort from the fact that the drug-abuse rate nationally in 1999 was coming down. "It's a cyclical problem," he says, driven by social forces that we, as a society, aren't good at analyzing or affecting.

Dr. Gaunt wishes that there was research data to underlie everything we say about effects of and treatments for prenatal drug exposure. He notes, however, that apparently valid recent research suggests that one in six babies nationally has been exposed to drugs. That finding is potentially frightening, but we have no research that clearly shows what it means. These babies "may be at risk for attention deficit, for example," but whether their intelligence or ability to reason is affected, either positively or negatively, we don't know.

The best we can say about treating the babies with the best care techniques we know is that, "These techniques are helpful. They help the baby during a transition period. If the baby had been in a dysfunctional environment instead, with inadequate feeding and overall neglect, the long-term impact could be severe. Good foster homes can provide the needed care, but the drug-affected baby is a little bit challenging: more demanding, fussier, more irritable, harder to feed. Parents and caregivers feel more comfortable with a center that can provide good care and advice drawn from their tremendous experience."

One might think that Dr. Gaunt's considerable experience with these babies might have attracted the attention of other pediatricians. He regrets that he has not had the time to write about the problems of and treatments for drug-affected babies. He'd rather spend the time with his patients, a choice that brings him great satisfaction but prevents him from being a research leader. His experience leads him to conclude that, even without documentation by research, the center's model of care needs to be exported to other parts of this country and the world, particularly to reduce the cost of hospital care (often about $2,500 per day, in contrast with the center's costs of $145 per day). He also cautions that getting enough hospital referrals may be the biggest obstacle to setting up other such centers.

DR. DAVID WOODRUM

As Professor of Neonatal and Respiratory Diseases, Pediatrics, University of Washington, Dr. David Woodrum serves as medical director of the neonatal intensive care unit at the University of Washington Hospital, with a specialty in high-risk pregnancies and new-

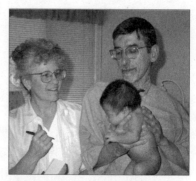

Dr. David Woodrum and Staff Nurse Kathleen Ewing.

born infants. He has over thirty years of experience as a pediatrician, though he limits his claim of expertise only to babies, not the long-term outcome of prenatal drug exposure.

A few years ago, when the media were raising fears about the perils of prenatal exposure to illegal drugs, he took an evening telephone call from an assistant to the mayor of Seattle. The caller said that Mayor Norm Rice and Rev. Jesse Jackson wanted to come to the University of Washington Hospital "to see some crack babies." He replied that there might be one or two who had been exposed to crack, "But they're not exciting to look at. They don't cause many acute problems." His point was that, contrary to media hype, crack or other illicit drugs may well cause subtle—or, later, perhaps not so subtle—disturbances in babies' vital systems, but, "It's hard to factor them out. The same woman who abuses cocaine probably abuses narcotics and alcohol and tobacco and has poor nutrition and enormous stress levels. Teasing out those threads continues to be a dilemma." In other words, during infancy a crack baby doesn't look a lot different from other babies.

While waiting for partial solutions to this complex medical and sociological problem, Dr. Woodrum decided to act on his knowledge of our center. He volunteered his services as an "itinerant pediatrician." We responded enthusiastically, pleased with the opportunity to have him share the burden—and the joy—with Dr. Gaunt. They rotate every other month, and he "thoroughly enjoys it."

He sees the existence of our center as "necessary because of the disorder that exists within drug-abusing families." Problems with finding adequate homes tend to prolong babies' stay at the center to an average of thirty-five days. But it is also true, he thinks, that care provided in our kind of center is preferable to care in a hospital—and not just for financial reasons. "In the absence of significant medical problems, the farther you can get from a hospital the better."

When asked about his position of breast-feeding the drug-exposed infant, Dr. Woodrum agrees that, given the present state of knowledge about the effects of drugs on breast milk, our policy of discouraging breast-feeding by these mothers is "a reasonable position." He also observes that drug-abusers often have the best of intentions, but "their psychological and physical needs sometimes make it hard for them to follow through on those intentions."

One of the most recent summaries of knowledge on the subject of breast-feeding is titled, *Medications and Mother's Milk* by Thomas Hale, (Pharmasoft Medical Publishing, 1999). It is a compilation of recommendations by the American Academy of Pediatrics (AAP) and of detailed evidence from recent studies. Following are excerpts from a few of these findings that pertain to drug use (both illicit and prescription) and breast-feeding:

DRUG	AAP RECOMMENDATION	PEDIATRIC CONCERNS
alcohol (ethanol)	Approved during breast-feeding though not during pregnancy.	If breast-fed within 2 to 3 hours after mother's drinking alcohol, infant may be sedated, irritable, or have weak suck (pp. 250-251).
amphetamines	Not approved.	Significant amounts of drug likely to transfer into milk, especially soon after mother's taking them; hallucinations, extreme agitation, and seizures likely; at least 24 hours between administration and breast-feeding needed to reduce risks significantly (pp. 48-49).
cocaine	Not approved.	Significant secretion into breast milk suspected, with significant agitation in infant resulting; extreme danger likely to infant (pp. 171-172).
haloperidol	No recommendation.	No concerns reported via milk, but caution recommended (p. 325).
heroin	Not approved.	Known to transfer to breast milk; detoxification preceding breast-feeding recommended (p. 337).
marijuana (cannabis)	Not approved.	Small to moderate secretion into breast milk documented, insufficient to produce significant side effects in infant; main concern is sedation (pp. 99-100).
methadone	Conditionally approved.	AAP recommendation based on dosage of 20 mg/24 hrs.; need to observe infant for sedation, respiratory depression, addiction, and withdrawal symptoms (pp. 449-450).
nicotine	Not reviewed.	Reduces milk production; no direct effects on infants reported but observe for shock, vomiting, diarrhea, rapid heart beat, and restlessness (pp. 503-504).

Dr. Woodrum's feelings for the babies he sees at the center are strong and, as he says, "humbling. At the outset of their lives, they already have greater burdens than most of us will have for our whole lives. The greatest of these burdens is the potential absence of security. Where will they go?" Dr. Woodrum noted that we have too few foster parents, and placement can be haphazard. He thinks we spend too few resources on choosing and training foster parents.

Another of the children's burdens is potential damage to cognitive capacity or intelligence. This is one of the more subtle long-term effects that Dr. Woodrum says has been impossible to "tease out" and quantify. He asserts that one cannot draw conclusions about intellect early in life (first several years). As for whether such children are likely to have ADHD (attention deficit hyperactivity disorder), no conclusions are possible until age six or seven. He goes further to suggest that, if you have a child who was prenatally exposed to drugs and is overly responsive to stimuli seven years later, "That is ADHD."

If research were to be done at our center, Dr. Woodrum doubts that it should focus on any of the "hard effects" of drugs on babies—their smartness or personalities or consolability. Rather, it should be a study of human interactions, with such questions as, "Can you teach excellent parenting?" The research would start at the center and follow the child into foster care or extended-family settings. If we took that path, we might get closer to solving a problem that is not primarily medical but social.

DR. ALVIN NOVACK

Formerly serving as head of the Division of General Pediatrics in the Department of Pediatrics, University of Washington School of Medicine, Dr. Alvin Novack is now partially retired. He was also medical director of the nursery at the University of Washington Medical Center, where he supervised care of drug-exposed infants, as well as normal (or "well") ones. Our association with him has been on committees related to the center.

In the 1980s, the University of Washington nursery cared for between fifty and eighty addicted newborns each year, with the goal—one that he fully supports—"to get these babies out of the hospital as soon as possible," well under the thirty-five-day average stay at our center. He, like Dr. Woodrum, believes that hospitals are not good places for babies, "even under the best of circumstances," and that our center is "much better than a hospital." Nevertheless, he also believes that two weeks is long enough for a withdrawing baby to be in a therapeutic-care setting.

Dr. Novack does not underestimate the potential dangers of withdrawal symptoms, particularly in babies who have been exposed to methadone. All babies have "very modest reserve capacities," he points out, meaning that they cannot go very long without feeding. When they do, they are in trouble, though he knows of no instances in which death resulted from withdrawal-caused lack of nutrition. If a baby undergoing withdrawal has both a poor suck and diarrhea "he or she can easily get into difficulty quickly. The potential for disease can be considerable, especially when the infant is premature and under normal weight."

Further complicating diagnosis and treatment of drug-exposed babies is the likelihood that, "They were exposed to substances that we don't know about—nicotine, alcohol, and other noxious things. There are methods of determining exposure to potentially toxic or harmful substances by analysis of babies' hair or meconium (first intestinal discharges of a newborn). Cocaine and other substances can be found there and, to a certain extent, it is possible to determine how much exposure occurred. But these methods are very expensive, and the information isn't all that helpful because we don't have therapeutic regimens to apply to the condition. It doesn't really pay, therefore, to go searching for that kind of information except in special circumstances."

As he explores alternatives to this kind of postnatal analysis, Dr. Novack shifts attention to the need for a drug-abusing mother's prenatal medical care. If she were receiving prenatal care and was found to be doing poorly, she might be hospitalized, assuming that she agreed. There, she would get adequate nutrition and, under supervision, decrease her intake of noxious substances.

In commenting on research done ten or more years ago, which seemed to show cause-and-effect relationships between a mother's prenatal drug use and behavioral symptoms in the infant, Dr. Novack dismisses much of the early research as "poor science." This research amounted to "horror stories"—that cocaine use, for example, results in specific congenital defects. Later studies, he said, tend to contradict this conclusion, leading him to believe that science cannot correlate prenatal use of a particular drug with certain symptoms, even if we could be sure that we had the means for knowing which drug or drugs the mother had used. Urine samples, for example, "are notoriously unreliable for determining exposure to short-acting substances."

He is also quick to say, "Cocaine is not good for a fetus. A fetus is much better off without it. But it is not as horrible as the media have made it seem. Alcohol and tobacco are much more damaging, at least from what we now know. Alcohol exposure during pregnancy has a long latent period, often showing up in teenagers. And cigarettes are highly implicated in a lot of different problems."

Dr. Novack says that the home environment that any drug-affected baby enters is the most important element in success or failure. If it includes parents with poor parenting skills, whether or not they are addicted, the effects on the child will almost certainly be negative. If the home is a truly nurturing environment, the child will do well. "This has been demonstrated very clearly in several studies. The fact that the baby went through withdrawal should have little significance on long-term outcome. That means that the baby will be neither any smarter nor any worse off than if there had been no prenatal drug exposure, though alcohol may be the exception to that generalization."

CONCLUSION

Since the Pediatric Interim Care Center opened, we have cared for more than 1,000 babies, and the oldest ones are now ten years old. All of our experience has shown us that it's the caregivers (mothers, fathers, grandparents, foster parents, teachers, day-care workers and social workers) who are the make-or-break factor in an infant's recovery and health.

Drug-exposed children have a bright future, but it hinges on the caregivers. We are not dealing with a throwaway generation. These children are beautiful, and they are like any other children—with good support at the beginning of their lives, they can bond and thrive. If they are given appropriate boundaries, reasonable discipline, routine, calm, and the sure knowledge that they are loved, they can cope very well. If their caregivers teach them how to manage their stimuli and environment, they seem to do just fine. These children are far more resilient than anyone previously thought. But it's the caregivers who give these children the tools they need to be resilient. The caregiver is the key to success.

GLOSSARY

The following terms are commonly used in therapeutic care of drug-exposed infants. All caregivers should be familiar with their meanings.

Attention Deficit Hyperactivity Disorder (ADHD)

A medical condition involving hyperactivity, often mistaken for the withdrawal effects of intrauterine drug exposure and often treated with the very drugs (such as Ritalin) that aggravate a drug-exposed child's symptoms.

Central Nervous System

The complex arrangement of nerves throughout the body that controls bodily functions.

Clapping

Rhythmic patting (to the beat of the adult's heart) of a swaddled and diapered infant's bottom.

Convulsion or Seizure

Generalized monoclonic jerks, involving more than one extremity.

C-Position

Placement of an infant's body so that it resembles the letter C (also known as fetal position).

Depressant

Any drug (such as alcohol, barbiturates, quaaludes, and tranquilizers) that acts on the central nervous system to produce both euphoria (feeling no pain) and drowsiness.

Disorganized Suck

Inability of an infant to latch on to nipple and suck regularly enough to get formula into the mouth.

Excoriation

Breakdown of skin resulting from rubbing against a surface.

Gastrointestinal

Relating to digestion in the stomach and intestines.

Gavage Feeding

Use of a naso-gastric tube, instead of a nippled bottle, to feed infants.

Hallucinogen

Any drug (such as marijuana, LSD, and PCP) that excites the brain, with the result that the user hallucinates, has mood changes, or even experiences short-term insanity.

Hypersensitivity

Greater than normal response to any stimulus (such as light, sound, and movement).

Inhalant
> Any substance (such as glue, nail polish remover, and gasoline) that, when inhaled, produces a high or feeling of euphoria.

Metabolism/Metabolic
> The processes of converting food to energy.

Myoclonic jerk
> Involuntary, quick, jerky muscle spasms involving one extremity at a time and much more noticeable than tremor.

Moro Reflex
> An indicator of hyperactivity or hypersensitivity.

Mottling
> Discoloration of skin resembling marbling, typically on chest, trunk, arms, or legs.

Muscle Tone
> The degree of rigidity in a muscle, associated with a muscle's ability to return to its original position when stretched.

Nasal Flaring
> Outward spreading of nostrils during breathing.

Neonatal Abstinence Scoring System

A tool that allows caregivers to observe and record signs and symptoms that indicate the withdrawal status of drug-exposed infants.

Opiates or Narcotic Analgesics

Any drug (such as opium, heroin, or methadone) that reduces the sensation of pain and induces a feeling of well-being.

Pediatric

Relating to the medical care of infants and young children.

Projectile Vomiting

Forceful vomiting of stomach contents.

Psychedelic

Any drug (such as LSD, peyote, or mescaline) that excites the brain, with the result that the user experiences strange visions or other distortions of reality.

Psychotropic

Any drug (such as Haloperidol, Chlorpromazine, or Thioridazine) that is prescribed by a doctor to treat a psychiatric disorder.

Regurgitation
Non-projectile vomiting of stomach contents.

Respiratory Rate
Speed of breathing.

Seizure or Convulsion
Generalized monoclonic jerks, involving more than one extremity.

Stimulant
Any drug (such as amphetamines, methamphetamines, cocaine, crack, or tobacco) that increases activity of the heart and provides an overall sense of well-being, at least temporarily.

Stool
Result of bowel movement; also called *feces*.

Swaddling
A method of folding a cotton-thermal blanket around an infant's body to restrain arm movement and give comfort.

Therapeutic Caregiver

    An adult male or female who provides specialized care for infants and young children who have been exposed before birth to powerful drugs (either prescribed, illegal, or not advised for pregnant women).

Therapeutic Handling

    Special techniques developed to care for drug-exposed infants.

Tremor

    Involuntary, rhythmical movements, resembling quivering, of a part of the body.

Vasomotor

    Relating to blood circulation.

Vertical Rock

    Up-and-down movement of an infant relative to the position of the standing or sitting adult who holds the infant.